HOW TO PREVENT FALLS

A Comprehensive Guide to Better Balance

By Betty Perkins-Carpenter

SENIOR FITNESS PRODUCTIONS

Rochester, New York

Published by: Senior Fitness Productions, Inc.
P.O. Box 25413
Rochester, New York 14625-2394

Printed in the United States of America

Second Edition

Library of Congress Catalog Card Number: 89-92153

Edited by Creative & Co.
Designed by 4D Advertising
Exercise illustrations by Bill Foley
Additional illustrations by Dick Roberts

ISBN 0-9621031-1-X

INTRODUCTION

"There is no doubt that elderly people can decrease the chance of serious injury and death from falls by taking steps to prevent them.

For several years, I have followed a regimen to help prevent falling. Now that I have read Betty Perkins-Carpenter's book, I have also begun the exercises that she describes.

I recommend this book to all…It should help significantly in reducing the probability of injury or death from falling."

Dr. Linus Pauling
Linus Pauling Institute
of Science and Medicine
Palo Alto, California

Dr. Linus Pauling is a world-renowned chemist, Nobel laureate and advocate of the use of Vitamin C for the prevention of illness.

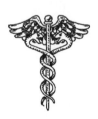

CONTENTS

CHAPTER 1: You Can Reduce The Risks Of Falling 1

CHAPTER 2: Don't Be Afraid To Be Fit 7

CHAPTER 3: Making The Balance System
Work For You 11

CHAPTER 4: The Balance System: Activities
For Better Balance...13

CHAPTER 5: Take It All In Stride:
Walking Toward Fitness................................77

APPENDIX 89

AFTERWORD 97

To my husband, who's one in a million, in all ways, always,
To my family, who have always believed in me,
To my staff, who held the fort, and
To all the wonderful seniors who trust me
and have faith in my work.

YOU CAN REDUCE
THE RISKS OF FALLING

**AMONG SENIORS,
FALLING IS THE
MOST COMMON,
LIFE-THREATENING
HAZARD**

Senior citizens represent the fastest growing segment of our nation's population. In fact, today there are actually more people over 65 than under 25. And for each and every one of these men and women, falling is the most common, life-threatening hazard.

Statistics gathered by the Center for Disease Control in 1988 indicated that among women between the ages of 65 and 85, falling is the second leading cause of death; among men in the same age group, it's the fourth. The risks of falling seem to increase dramatically with age. For those over the age of 85, falling is the leading cause of death!

**FALLS FALL INTO
TWO CATEGORIES**

Recent studies separate falls into two categories--those caused by external conditions and those caused by internal conditions. The external factors, such as poor lighting or scatter rugs, are simply easier to control than the internal factors.

Of the internal factors, physicians at the Yale University School of Medicine focus on five areas of vulnerability that contribute to falling: mental changes (such as confusion or dementia), circulatory problems (such as the inability of blood pressure to adjust to sudden changes in posture), gait or balance problems, medications (particularly sedatives), diseases (such as arthritis and osteoporosis), poor distance vision and, finally, muscular weakness.

FALLING IS NOT SIMPLY PART OF GROWING OLD

For years we took for granted that falling was simply part of growing old. True, aging **does** impose certain limitations on our bodies. The loss of some flexibility over the years (resulting from the loss of a natural substance called "elastin") is common. And, according to Dr. W. J. Evans, chief of the physiology laboratory at the Human Research Nutrition Center at Tufts, inactivity exacerbates the problem. Evans believes that most falls are "due to profound muscle weakness from not doing anything." Now, that's an opportunity for change!

By practicing and repeating certain movements on a regular basis, we can strengthen muscles that

2

have become inactive. Muscular strength is necessary for correction of balance errors. I agree with Bob Anderson, a fitness expert, when he says that "all of us have this seemingly miraculous capacity for regaining health, whether it be from something as drastic as surgery, or from poor physical condition caused by lack of activity and bad diet."

I know Bob is right. I work with seniors in a variety of settings, using what I call "The Balance System." **In every case**, their balance has improved. And although some of them have sustained accidental falls, **not one has been seriously hurt**! Improved balance **can** reduce the incidence of falling, as well as the resultant injuries!

THE BALANCE SYSTEM IMPROVES BOTH PHYSICAL AND EMOTIONAL WELL-BEING

What is The Balance System? It is a program that concentrates on both your physical and your emotional well-being. As you read through these chapters, you will find a variety of activities which were designed to promote muscle tone and balance. You will also find what I hope are appropriate reasons for why you **can** and **should** set aside your fears and get moving. The net result will be a new you--someone who has overcome the apprehension that has prevented him from revitalizing his life.

It's never too late to enhance or extend your capabilities. Age is not a factor. Why, some of my students are in their late nineties. One gentleman, whose accomplishments and enthusiasm are truly inspirational, has even mastered walking the "balance beam" (parallel strips of masking tape set out on the floor). When he started, he moved slowly from one end of the "beam" to the other, relying heavily on his walker. Now he traverses the beam quite proficiently, first lifting the walker right off the ground and now setting it aside!

Many seniors have had similar results time and time again. You **can** slow down the physical, mental and social deterioration that come with aging. You can exercise some control over the quality of your life. You can call back the years, feel pride in the development of new skills and in the power of your own competence.

OVERCOMING FEAR IS THE FIRST STEP I have also learned from the seniors I work with that fear is one of the primary obstacles in practicing to regain and improve their balance.

Dr. Richard Sattin, Chief of the Unintentional Injuries Section of the Center for Disease Control, agrees. "Many people who have fallen or who have seen their friends fall, develop a fear of falling. This can significantly affect their quality of life and threaten their ability to live independently."

With the right amount of determination and practice, though, you can meet your fears head-on and overcome them. Why, pretty soon what you thought was impossible will become FUN. You'll enjoy practicing your balance activities. And soon you'll find that you have conquered your fears!

2

DON'T BE AFRAID TO BE FIT

In my work with seniors, I've found that their own fears, real or imagined, are the major stumbling blocks to general fitness. Seniors are afraid to move, exercise or even attempt some of the simple Balance System movements for fear they might overdo or break something. Their reasoning is that moving an area which may already be weakened or strained could make it worse, and that it's better to conserve whatever mobility there is.

Fear **is** a stiff competitor. Fear contributes to feeling inadequate and insecure. There is no question that the result of falling is PAIN, and even thinking about falling is SCARY. This, coupled with the fact that most seniors are inclined to be tense and hold their bodies very tight, contributes to the high incidence of injuries resulting from falls.

According to sports psychologist Dr. Alan Goldberg, fear may be caused by not knowing what your body is doing in space. Dr. Goldberg suggests that "the MORE time you put into those (physical activities that scare you), the LESS scary they become."

Further studies at the Durham Veterans Hospital indicate that the attitude of elderly people toward accidents compounds the problem--seniors try to reduce the risk of injury by avoiding any situations that might result in a fall. Thus, many seniors choose not to move, and though inactivity does reduce the immediate risk of falling, its long term effects are just the opposite. **Movement is the key**. And balance is the basis for all movement.

In fact, the closest thing to an anti-aging pill is moving. It's true. Use favors function; disuse invites decay. And as I have described in **The Fun of Fitness**, the benefits of exercise and fitness go far beyond helping to reduce the risk of accidents or to encourage spatial awareness. Movement, activity and even exercise promote and enhance your mental, emotional and social well-being. Furthermore, they can make significant inroads toward relieving heart disease, arthritis, osteoporosis, obesity, high blood pressure and diabetes.

Those of you who have already followed the

recommendations in **The Fun of Fitness** know that exercise also contributes to improved eye-hand-foot coordination and to improved gross and fine motor skills. Reaction time improves, too. As movement enhances spatial awareness, so, too, does it enhance posture, poise and grace. And exercise causes the blood to carry more oxygen to the brain, which serves to increase the efficiency of the mind as well as the body! The overall effect, then, is to reduce stress and to improve your emotional outlook by increasing your confidence and self-esteem.

The better you feel, the more you want to share your good fortune with others. Fitness and sociability can support each other. You may find that using The Balance System with a partner or in a group helps to establish and reinforce a routine. So be sure and plan to share The Balance System with a friend!

There are no guarantees that we will never have an accident or that we can prevent an unforeseen fall, but we can be physically and mentally prepared for reducing the risks. How? First, take steps to control the elements in your environment that increase the likelihood of falls. (I have included my recommendations for reducing the external risks in the Appendix to this booklet.) Then, talk with your doctor, set realistic goals, track your progress, and don't be discouraged if you don't master a task at once. Just keep trying. But start today. Don't let fear get in your way. Remember, safe adults are no accident!

MAKING THE BALANCE SYSTEM WORK FOR YOU

Please, before you begin any exercise or movement program, check with your physician to be sure which activities are appropriate for you. And have your doctor help you set realistic goals. Aim high, but set your sights within the range of your capabilities. Listen to your body. As you get stronger, it will help confirm your progress. If you're overdoing it, those aches and pains are telling you to slow down a little. (Yes, there **can** be gain without pain!)

Beyond setting balance and fitness goals, I have found setting certain other goals useful in the success of any activity program.

First, **set aside a specific time of day for your balance activities**. Make them part of your routine. For instance, before you brush your teeth or before your first morning cup of coffee, before lunch or dinner, reserve just a few minutes for at least one or two Balance System activities. And, as I mentioned before, you might find that sharing the activities with a friend or group can help you establish your routine. (Plus, it's more fun!)

Second, **stay with it**. There's no substitute for practice. We all know that the more frequently we do something--anything, from practicing a musical instrument to golf--the better we become. Perseverance pays off!

Third, **keep a good mental outlook**. A positive attitude reinforces the determination that, while we may not be twenty years old or great athletes, maintaining the muscular strength we need to correct balance errors can help us be fit. Again, it's just a matter of starting slowly and practicing the activities regularly.

By using the activities in The Balance System, you are providing yourself with an opportunity to improve both your fitness and the quality of your life. Don't be afraid to start. And, then, when your well-meaning children or friends gasp and tell you "you shouldn't do that," you can simply smile and say, "not only **should** I ... I **can**."

4

THE BALANCE SYSTEM:
ACTIVITIES FOR BETTER BALANCE

The following series of activities is designed to promote both your balance awareness and your balance ability. The activities have been grouped to take you on a comfortable journey from simple, "getting started" movements to balance movements that are progressively more advanced.

Although many of these Balance System activities require no special equipment, some do call for the use of simple "props," such as a chair, a bed or a "balance beam" (which you can make by placing parallel lengths of masking tape right on your floor).

Before you try any of The Balance System activities, familiarize yourself with your balance point and a few simple warm-up activities.

FIND YOUR BALANCE POINT

You'll find that the majority of Balance System activities ask you to begin by finding your "balance point." Because we are all unique, we each have our own balance point or center of gravity. By this I mean the position in which, when you are balancing, your weight is evenly distributed and you feel comfortable and safe. Here's how to find your own, individual balance point.

Ideally, if you dropped a plumb line down from your head through the center of your body, you'd find your "center of balance," the position in which you'd feel most balanced (secure) and least likely to fall.

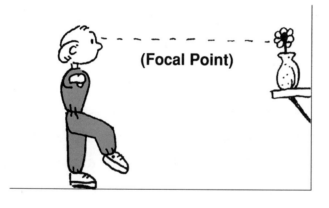

(Focal Point)

One tip that you may find helpful in establishing your **own** balance point is to keep your eyes set on a fixed point. Whether you're focusing on a mark on the floor, a crack in the wall or a television set across the room, keeping your eyes on one spot, or what I call your "focal point," will help you to concentrate more fully on **feeling** your balance.

As you can see from the illustrations, there are several positions in which you may be most comfortable balancing. Try doing so with:

14

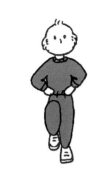

1.

- your hands on your hips;

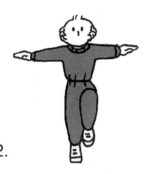

2.

- your arms outstretched to the sides like a telephone pole;

> For practical purposes (and since most people use this position), Balance System activities illustrate the balance point with arms extended to the sides at shoulder level as in illustration #2.

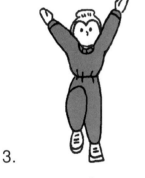

3.

- your arms raised in a "V" position;

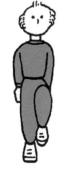

4.

- your arms at your sides.

Whatever your position, be sure you feel comfortable and safe. Become aware of your balance point. Practice it, and let it become second nature to you **before** you begin your Balance System activities.

WARM UP TO ELIMINATE STRAINED MUSCLES

The longer you go without using certain muscles, the shorter those muscles eventually become. This muscle "shrinkage" means that even the slightest over-exertion (sometimes your activities program itself) can create real problems. That's why nearly every fitness plan recommends warming up before exercising.

Just as its name suggests, this preliminary activity literally warms up the muscles to make them more pliable and resilient

The best muscle warmer of all is your own circulation. And moderate exercising brings the blood slowly to your muscles, warming them gradually and preparing them properly for the exercises ahead.

You can warm up first by stretching. Stretching:

- increases your range of motion;
- decreases your risks of injury/muscle strains;
- promotes better circulation;
- improves your flexibility, so you can be more active with greater ease;
- improves your energy level.

Stretching should not be painful. Stretch according to how it feels to **you**. Breathe slowly and rhythmically; never hold your breath. Stretch gently and slowly, feeling a mild tension in your muscles. Now, try these techniques on the following warm-up activities.

Listen to your own body and do only what is comfortable to you.

TRY THESE WARM-UPS BEFORE STARTING YOUR BALANCE SYSTEM ACTIVITIES.

SHAKE IT UP AND STRETCH IT OUT

Here's a super-stretcher that will get your whole body feeling loose and relaxed!

FOR STARTERS: Stand tall, with your feet comfortably together, arms loosely at your sides.

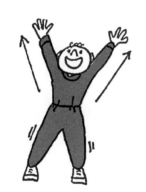

1. Stretch your arms up over your head, then stretch them out to the sides and stretch your fingertips down toward the floor.
2. Now, RELAX. Try to feel an overall "looseness," as if your arms and whole body were "cooked spaghetti"--face, eyes, lips, neck and so on, right down to your toes. (Let go. As they say in Hawaii, "hang loose.")

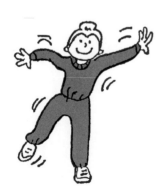

3. Next, shake your loose right arm. Shake your loose left arm.
4. Shake your loose right leg, then your loose left leg.
5. Now, wiggle your "okole" (from Hawaii again, that's the word for buttocks).
6. Keep moving your arms, legs and buttocks until you feel completely loose and relaxed.

Whenever you warm up or do any of your Balance System activities, stand as tall as you possibly can, with your shoulders square and your chest up.

•   Be sure to feel comfortable with each step before proceeding to the next.

•   To increase the tactile stimulation to your feet, practice in your bare or stocking feet. Sneakers are fine if you prefer. Just avoid wearing socks or smooth-soled shoes or slippers on wood or waxed floors.

ELEVATOR GOING UP (AND DOWN)

Our legs seem to be the first "trouble spot" of our anatomy. We need to keep them as strong as possible, though, for mobility, equilibrium and balance.

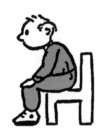

FOR STARTERS: Sit in a stationary chair. Feet should be a comfortable distance apart and arms should be at your sides, or hands resting on your knees or thighs, whichever is best for you.

Make believe you are on an elevator going up one floor at a time and stopping (holding your position) for a few seconds at each floor. Let's use a four-story building.

1. Stand up a little and hold: first floor.

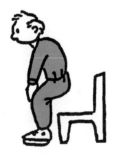

2. Stand up a little further and hold: second floor.
3. Stand up further still and hold: third floor.

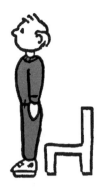

4. Now stand up tall as the elevator reaches the top (4th) floor.
5. Repeat, coming back down to a sitting position. Hold at each floor as you return to your starting position, sitting comfortably in your chair.

Do this activity every day to increase muscle strength in your legs.

FITNOTE   I'll bet very few of us pay much attention to our feet. But there are muscles on the top and the bottom of the foot. And those muscles can be protected against injury simply by warming them up before practicing any balance activities. Here are a few warm-up activities for your feet, which, incidentally, also help to prevent sprained ankles.

- Spread toes out and curl them up. Always try to maintain your ability to open and close your toes.
- Play games with your toes. With bare feet, try to pick up marbles and move them from one spot to another. Pick up your shoe lace, place it on top of your shoe, then move it back to the floor.
- "Lift" your arch, then toes, then heels up off the floor.
- Massage your feet and each toe, using your thumbs.

BAREFOOT IN THE PARK

Actually, you don't have to set foot outside the house, just "park it" on the floor or bed and see how good your feet and legs feel with this one.

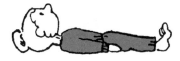 **FOR STARTERS:** Lie flat on the floor, in bed, or sit tall in a chair.

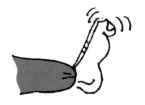

1. Curl and tense your toes as tightly as you can. Hold for a slow count of 1 – 2 – 3, then uncurl and relax.

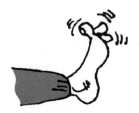

2. Next, wiggle your toes and relax.

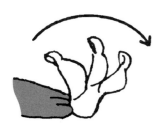

3. Now, "flutter" your feet one at a time (like you would your eyelashes).

4. Relax and "shake out" your feet.

REPETITIONS: 8 times, each foot.

FITNOTE Your feet will feel great when held under COLD running water. Or, soak them in HOT water, then cold, hot and finish with cold.

TOOTSIES ROLL

PROP: Rolling pin

FOR STARTERS: Stand (preferably) or sit tall, with bare feet.

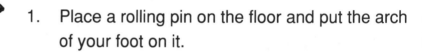

1. Place a rolling pin on the floor and put the arch of your foot on it.

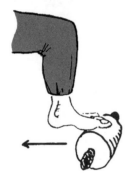

2. Now, slowly roll your foot backwards over the pin (to the tips of your toes). Then roll your foot all the way to your heel. Apply pressure to the pin as you move your foot. (You'll feel how much pressure to apply.)

3. Repeat the rolling movements with your other foot. (Always exercise both feet, even if you think only one foot needs it.)

REPETITIONS: 2 to 3 times

HINT: If you do this one while standing, please be sure to hold on to the back of a straight chair or counter for balance and safety.

The National Council on Aging's most recent research proves that maintaining strength in ankles, feet and toes is crucial to better balance.

ONE FOR THE BOOKS

You'll need a telephone book (or favorite novel) for this one! No reading involved...just good strengthening of ankles and feet.

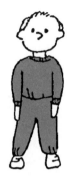

PROP: Book

FOR STARTERS: Stand tall, with feet slightly apart on the floor. As an alternative, try this exercise sitting down.

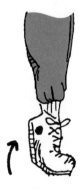

1. Slowly raise both heels until your weight is on the balls of your feet. Hold for a count of 1 – 2 – 3. Lower and relax. Repeat 5 to 10 times.

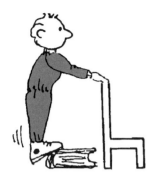

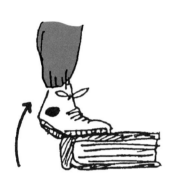

2. Now position the book on the floor so that the binding is facing you.

3. Hold on to the back of a straight chair and with the front half of your feet, step up onto the book. Slowly raise both heels until your weight is on the balls of your feet. Hold for a count of 1 – 2 – 3. Lower and relax.

4. Repeat 5 to 10 times.

REPETITIONS: Do series 1 to 2 times

ADVANCED VERSION

Once you've mastered the phone book, you can try it on the bottom stair, holding on to the railing for balance. For an even more advanced method, go back to the phone book and this time when you raise and lower your heels, stop every 2 inches, holding each position for 3 counts.

THE BALANCE SYSTEM ACTIVITIES

Now that you're all warmed up and ready to go, try a few of The Balance System activities found on the following pages. Start with the easiest ones, which come first in order, and SLOWLY move on to the more advanced movements.

Don't attempt to do them all at once! For some seniors it might take eight to twelve weeks or more to get through the whole set. Don't be discouraged. Work at your own, most relaxed pace. Then, when you've tried each of them, work out your own routine of favorites. And remember, you can do it. Yes, you can!

FIRST STEPS

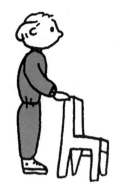

FOR STARTERS: Stand tall with feet slightly apart. Rest your right hand on the back of a stationary chair beside you. **Or**, place both hands on the back of a stationary chair in front of you.

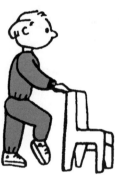

1. Holding onto the chair, raise your right knee so your foot is a few inches off the floor. (Higher once you've mastered the movements.) Allow your right leg, from knee to foot, to hang loose. (Be careful not to tuck your foot under your thigh!) Hold this position for a count of 1 – 2 – 3.
2. Return right leg to starting position and relax.
3. Repeat the activity with your left leg.

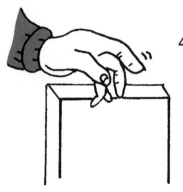

4. Now, "play the piano" by rippling your fingertips on the back of the chair. (By this I mean practice how it feels to balance without the complete support of the chair.)

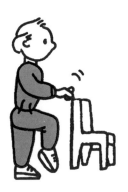

5. While "playing piano," repeat lifting your right knee and then your left knee (steps 1, 2 & 3 on the previous page) just high enough to sense how it might feel to completely let go of the chair.

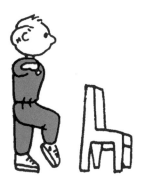

6. Now, raise your right knee so that your foot is a few inches off the floor. Slowly (and RELAXED) let go of the chair and gently raise your arms, little by little, until you find your balance point. Hold this position as long as you can. (At first, it might be just a fraction of a second, but gradually you will be able to hold your position for longer intervals.)

7. Return your hands to the chair and lower your right leg. RELAX.

8. Repeat with your left leg.

REPETITIONS: As many as you enjoy!

HINT: Experiment with the positions described in BALANCE POINTS.

CHORUS LINE

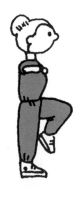

FOR STARTERS: Stand tall, feet together, and arms at your balance point.

1.   Lift your left knee so that your foot is just off the floor.

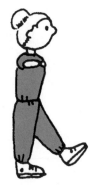

2.   Straighten your left leg out in front of you.

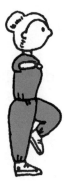

3.   Return to bent-knee position and lower left foot to the floor.
4.   Relax and repeat activity using your right leg.

REPETITIONS: 2 sets (a set equals right and left leg).

ADVANCED VERSION

1. When your leg is straightened in Step 2, point your toes and really s – t – r – e – t – c – h.
2. Hold the stretch for a count of 1 – 2 – 3. FEEL those leg muscles work!
3. Gently "push" your heel forward toward the floor. Hold for a count of 1 – 2 – 3.
4. Flex your ankle to bring your toes up toward your body, then down, away from your body.
5. Gently, with the ankle very loose and relaxed, rotate your ankle clockwise and then counter-clockwise.

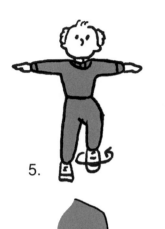

5.

REPETITIONS: Do as many as you enjoy.

FITNOTE

You may get cramps from stretching. If you do, drink lots of water, as you could be a bit dehydrated. If cramp persists, "knead" it like you would bread dough.

HEEL-TO-TOE

FOR STARTERS: Stand tall, feet slightly apart and arms at balance point.

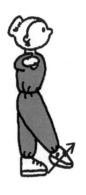

1. Relax and then raise your right leg straight out in front of you, with your foot just off the floor.

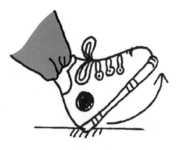

2. Now, touch your heel to the floor, then touch your toes to the floor. Repeat heel-to-toe touching 4 times.

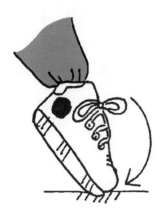

3.   Lower right leg and relax.

4.   Repeat the activity with your left leg.

REPETITIONS: 2 or 3 times.

A D V A N C E D   V E R S I O N

Do not allow heel or toe to touch floor. Flex your ankle and do **Heel-To-Toe** "in the air."

FITNOTE   It takes time to build your self-confidence. Be delighted with every improvement because you know it means you're reducing the risk of a fall!

A REAL SWINGER

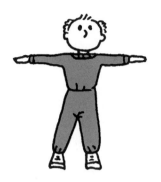

FOR STARTERS: Stand tall, feet slightly apart, arms at your balance point.

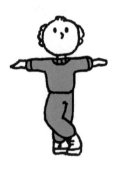

1. Bend your right knee and cross your right foot in front of and to the outside of your left foot, touching your right toes to the floor.

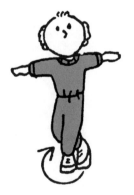

2. With knee still bent, gently swing your right leg from the front position to behind your left leg, touching your right toes to the floor.

3. Return to starting position, relax and repeat activity using your left leg.

REPETITIONS: 4 times with right leg and then 4 times with left leg. You may enjoy 1 time, right leg and then 1 time, left leg. Your choice!

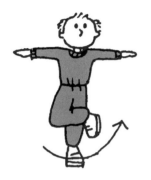

ADVANCED VERSION

Practice being **A Real Swinger** without touching toes to the floor! Gently "swing" the leg front and back, front and back. Then, move foot in front, out to the side and behind.

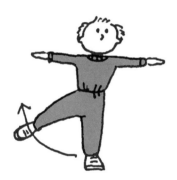

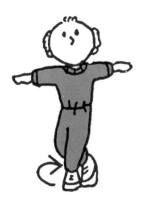

SWING TIME

FOR STARTERS: Stand tall, feet slightly apart and arms at your balance point.

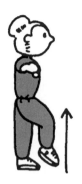

1. Lift your right knee so that your foot is comfortably off the floor.

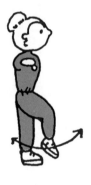

2. Gently swing your lower leg, from the knee to the foot, forward and backward like, a pendulum, 5 times.

3. Lower your leg and relax.

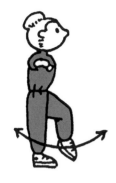

4.   Repeat the activity with your left leg.

REPETITIONS: Alternating your right and left legs, repeat steps 1-3 as many times as you wish.

FITNOTE Remember, **in all your balance activities**, as you hold your arms up in your balance position, you are increasing your arm strength and endurance.

FLAMINGO DANCE

FOR STARTERS: Stand tall, feet slightly apart and arms at balance point.

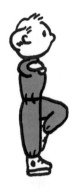

1. Raise your left knee and place your left foot on the inside of your right calf. Hold for a count of 1 – 2 – 3.

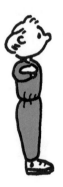

2. Now, slowly slide your left foot back to the floor.

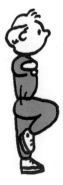

3. Relax, then repeat activity using your right foot.

REPETITIONS: Alternating legs 3 to 4 times.

ADVANCED VERSION

You can increase the difficulty of **Flamingo Dance** by lifting your foot higher and resting it on the inside of the knee. Then slowly slide your foot down to the calf; stop and hold for a count of 1 – 2 – 3; lower to ankle and hold for a count of 1– 2 – 3; then back to the floor. Repeat with other foot.

BALANCE BALLET

FOR STARTERS: Stand tall, feet slightly apart and arms at balance point.

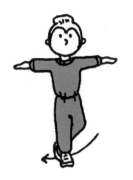

1.   Bend your left knee and bring your left leg behind your right leg, so that the left leg is resting low on the right calf, toes on the floor.

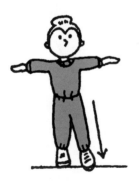

2.   Bring your left leg around to the starting position and stretch it out in front of you with toes pointed down, just above the floor.

3.   Return to the starting position and relax.

4.   Repeat the activity using your right leg.

REPETITIONS: 2 sets (a set being right and left legs).

ADVANCED VERSIONS

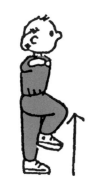

Challenge yourself! Repeat steps 1 and 2 a total of 4 times without touching the floor.

SIDESTEPPING

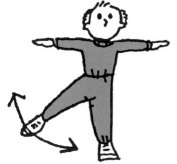

1. Lift your right knee up and then straighten your right leg out to the side.
2. Gently swing it up and down 2 or 3 times. Repeat with left leg.

REPETITIONS: 1 or 2 times

FLYAWAY

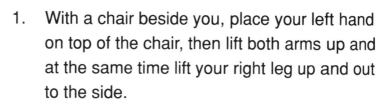

1. With a chair beside you, place your left hand on top of the chair, then lift both arms up and at the same time lift your right leg up and out to the side.
2. Lower your arms and right leg, and repeat using left leg.

When you feel comfortable and secure, then do the **Flyaway** without a chair.

REPETITIONS: 2 or 3 times

RAISE YOUR HAND

FOR STARTERS: Stand tall, feet slightly apart and arms at balance point.

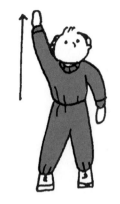

1.

1. Stretch your right arm over your head as far as is comfortable for you.

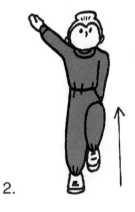

2.

2. With right arm still extended, raise your left knee as high as you comfortably can.

3. Lower your right arm and left leg and relax.

4. Repeat the activity using the left arm and right leg.

REPETITIONS: Repeat 2 or 3 times.

ADVANCED VERSION

1. Raise your right arm over your head and, at the same time, raise your left knee.

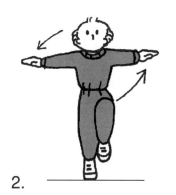

2.   2. Holding that position, lower right arm and raise left arm until both arms are at shoulder level.

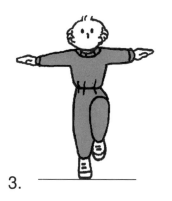

3.   3. Now, straighten the left leg out to the front without touching the floor; hold for a count of 3, bend knee, lower leg and relax.

4. Lower arms and relax.
5. Repeat using the left arm and right leg.

REPETITIONS: As many as you enjoy!

THE BALANCE BEAM

Before proceeding to the following balance activities, make yourself a "balance beam" to practice on as you go about your daily routine. Since we don't have regulation beams in our homes, we have to be creative and make our own!

Simply lay down strips of masking tape about 8' long on a rug or on the floor. Depending on the width of your tape, you will put down 2 to 4 strips, side by side, so that your "beam" is 4" wide.

4" wide {
————————————————————
————————————————————
————————————————————

(Remember to place your "beam" in an area you use frequently. The more you practice, the safer you'll be!)

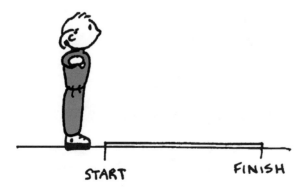

START   FINISH

TIGHTROPE WALKER

FOR STARTERS: Stand comfortably in front of your masking tape "balance beam."

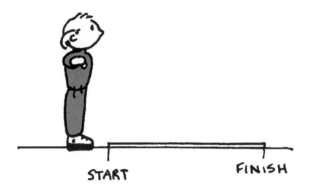

START   FINISH

1. Hold your arms out horizontally, at shoulder level, just like a tightrope walker. Feel relaxed.
2. Stepping very slowly (without running down the "beam"), place one foot in front of the other on the "beam." It doesn't matter which foot you start with, but do try to space your feet about 4" apart (between the heel of the leading foot and the toe of the trailing foot) and feel in good balance. You should try to walk normally, but you might want to experiment turning your toes out and your heels in a bit for better balance. Just be sure to feel your balance point before going on.

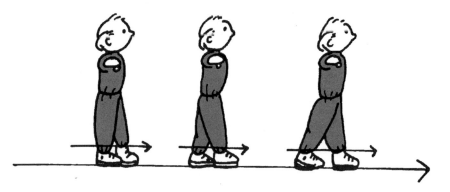

3. Continue walking along the "beam." Your eyes should focus on the end of the "beam" (or 3 or 4 feet in front of you or on a target straight ahead, at eye level). Just DON'T look down at your feet!

4. Walk to the end of the "beam" with a slow, normal gait, staying on the parallel taped lines and maintaining your feel for balance with each step. If you're barefoot, in socks or stockings, FEEL the tape with your toes. Sensory perception in our feet is very important to balance.

5. When you reach the end, lower your arms and relax. Now, turn around and walk the "beam" back. (As you turn, focus your eyes straight ahead.) Maintain good posture, shoulders back, chest up.

REPETITIONS: As many as you enjoy doing!

If you have an extreme fear of falling, you may wish to start with the following variations.

1. Place your right foot on the tape and your left foot off the tape and walk normally to the end. Turn and come back with your left foot on the tape and your right foot off.
2. Stand with both feet on the tape and move your right foot forward and bring your left foot to meet your right foot – step forward – close – step forward – close.
3. Stand on tape facing sideways and slowly slide your right foot to the right and bring left foot to meet right foot. Slide sideways to the right and return sliding sideways to the left.

ADVANCED VERSION

When you've mastered the fine art of "tightrope walking" forward, you might want to try it backwards. I can hear you now! "I can't do that!" Yes, you can. In fact, you may also walk sideways, known as "sidestepping."

Or, try "crossovers." Cross your left foot over your right, going to the right on the "beam." Then cross right over left on your return trip.

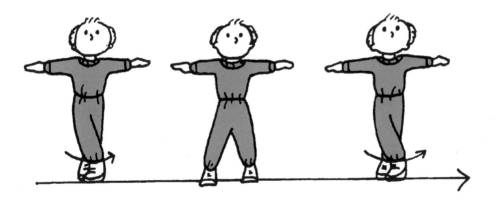

Feeling really confident? Walk on your toes! Yes, you can!

PEDALER'S POISE

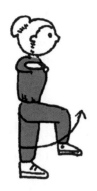

1.

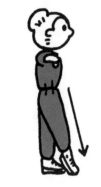

2a.

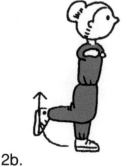

2b.

FOR STARTERS: Stand tall, feet slightly apart and arms at your balance point.

1. Raise your right knee, putting your foot on a make-believe bicycle pedal, just off the floor.

2. Start to "pedal" (2a and 2b) by moving your right foot in a downward, circular path and brushing the floor with your toes. (Remember to point your toes down, just as you would on a real bike pedal. This is also great for increasing your ankle flexibility!)

3. Return your right foot to the floor and relax.

4. Repeat the activity using your left leg.

REPETITIONS: 3 rotations each leg.

ADVANCED VERSIONS

Don't touch the floor with your toes! Then, increase the degree of difficulty by lifting your knee higher and higher off the floor, making larger circles with your "pedaling" motion. Also go in reverse! Pedal backwards.

VARIATIONS:

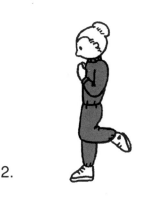

2.

1. Close your eyes during **Pedaler's Poise**.
2. Place your hands in a praying position in front of your chest, fingers pointed toward the ceiling. Drop your head gently, chin toward chest. Close your eyes. Bend one knee and lift your heel toward your buttocks. Try to hold your balance while counting slowly to 5, then work up to 10 and beyond.

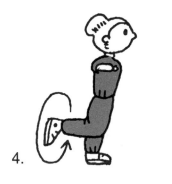

4.

3. Bend your right knee and gently place the toes of your right foot on the floor behind you. (I call this variation the **Slow Back Spin**.)
4. Lift your right heel up toward your buttocks and move your toes in a small, slow, gentle circle, first clockwise and then counter-clockwise.
5. Lower foot to floor and repeat with left leg. Relax.

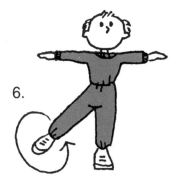

6.

6. LIft your right leg out to the side and complete 2 small circles clockwise.
7. Lower leg and relax.
8. Repeat using your left leg. I call this activity the **Side-Winder**.

REPETITIONS: 1 or 2 times

YOU'RE IN THE ARMY NOW

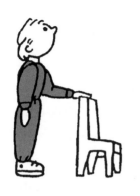

FOR STARTERS: Stand tall, with your feet slightly apart and your hand resting on a stationary chair in front of you. Ten-hut, soldier, it's march time!

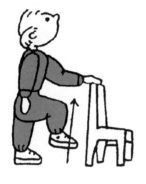

1. Holding onto the back of the chair for support, alternate lifting your right knee then your left. March in place for a count of 1 – 2…1 – 2 – 3 1 – 2…1 – 2 – 3, etc.

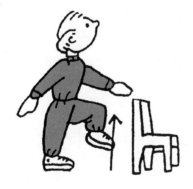

2. Now, still marching, slowly let go of the chair. Find your balance point. Try swinging your arms to the rhythm of your feet. March in place.

REPETITIONS: 30 seconds to 1 minute and gradually increase endurance.

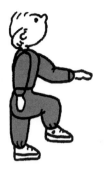

ADVANCED VERSION

Move away from the chair. Really swing those arms! March as if you were in the army, and then, as your left arm and right leg lift up – stop – and hold them both up momentarily, then lower your arm and leg and march again. Repeat by holding right arm and left leg up momentarily. (As you gently swing your arms, you are maintaining your shoulder flexibility, arm strength and endurance.)

TAP DANCE

FOR STARTERS: Stand tall, feet slightly apart and arms at your balance point.

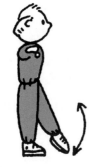

1. & 2.

1. Raise your left leg straight out in front of you, so that your foot is just off the floor, toes pointed.
2. Move your leg up and down, tapping your toes to the floor 3 times.

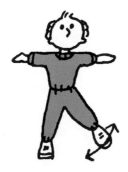

3. Now, move your left leg out to the side, with your foot just off the floor, and tap 3 times.

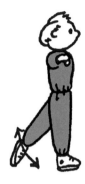

4. Continue to move your left leg around behind you, and tap 3 times.

5. Return to starting position and relax.
6. Repeat activity using your right leg.

REPETITIONS: 2 sets (1 set is right and left legs).

ADVANCED VERSION

To increase the difficulty, don't touch the floor while "tapping."

BALANCING ACT

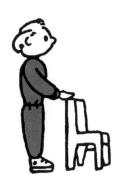

FOR STARTERS: Stand tall, hands resting on a stationary chair in front of you.

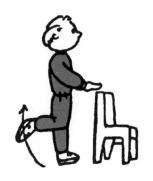

1. With both hands on the chair, bend your right leg at the knee so that your foot is behind you.

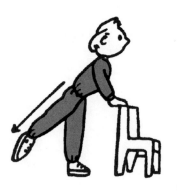

2. Lean slightly forward toward the chair. Straighten your right leg out behind you to a comfortable position and gently point your toes.
3. Then bend your knee. Return to starting position and relax.
4. Repeat the activity with your left leg. (Be sure you have become comfortable with steps 1 – 4 before going on to next page!)

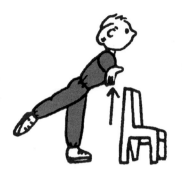

5. "Play the piano" on the chair with your fingertips and slowly raise your arms to your balance point. Extend your right leg out behind you as you lean toward the chair. Hold for a count of 1 – 2 – 3.

6. Return to the start of step 5 and repeat using your left leg.

7. Now, move your feet a little further away from the chair and repeat steps 5 and 6.

REPETITIONS: As often as you can.

Remember, if you feel yourself losing your balance, just place your hands back onto the chair to steady yourself.

TIPSY
(SIDEWARD MOVEMENT)

FOR STARTERS: Sit up tall in an armless chair.

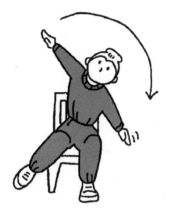

1. Put arms out to side at shoulder height.
2. Lift up right knee and slowly tip to the left as you straighten right leg out to side and slightly forward.
3. Tip as far as you safely can. Slowly return to sitting position, bend knee and place foot back on the floor.

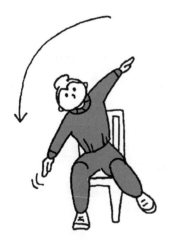

4. Repeat to right side lifting and straightening left leg.

REPETITIONS: As often as possible.

FITNOTE

For fun, and between repetitions, practice **"Upsa-Daisy."** Stand up, sit down, stand up, turn around and sit down. When you feel safe and secure doing this activity, close your eyes as you stand up, turn around and sit down. Quite a different feeling!

STEADY AS SHE GOES

FOR STARTERS: Stand tall, feet slightly apart, with your left hand resting on a stationary chair beside you.

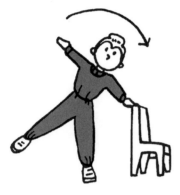

1. With left hand on the chair, raise your right leg out to the side and your right arm to a comfortable balance point.
2. Hold the position for a count of 5. **Steady as she goes**!
3. Return to starting position and relax.

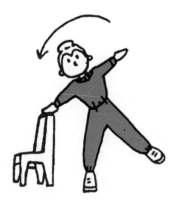

4. Repeat the activity with your right hand on chair and using your left leg and arm.

REPETITIONS: Right and left as a series, three times.

63

HIP HIP HOORAY!

Hip Hip Hooray! is a very advanced balance activity. Be sure you are experienced and feel safe and secure with all the other balance activities before proceeding to **Hip Hip Hooray!**. The first time you try these movements, you may wish to use a chair that has been placed against a wall so it cannot move.

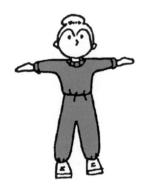

FOR STARTERS: Stand tall, feet slightly apart, arms at your balance point.

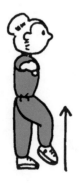

1. Lift your right knee so your foot is just off the floor.

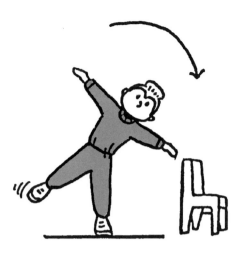

2. Lean a little bit to the left while straightening your right leg to the side for balance. Remember not to lift your right leg too high, just barely off the floor.

3. Bend your knee again as you return to your starting position.

4. Now repeat the routine with your left leg, while leaning to the right.

REPETITIONS: As many as you can.

LEAN INTO IT

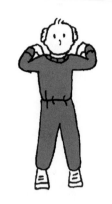

FOR STARTERS: Stand tall, hands resting on your shoulders.

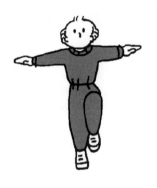

1. Simultaneously, bring left knee up and move arms out to shoulder level.

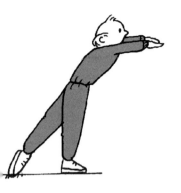

2. Slowly lean forward as your left leg stretches out behind you and both hands reach out in front of you.

3. The first time you do the exercise (or until you feel comfortable) rest your left foot on the floor behind you.

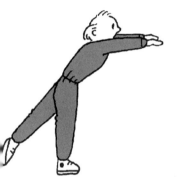

4. When you feel comfortable with the exercise, lift your foot off the floor.

SPIN CYCLE

FOR STARTERS: Stand tall, feet slightly apart and arms at sides.

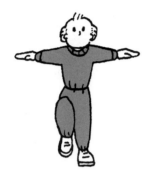

1.   Raise your right knee so your foot is just off the floor.

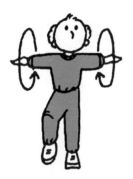

2.   Lift your arms out to the side at shoulder level and trace small clockwise circles in the air.
3.   Lower your right leg and arms and relax.
4.   Using your left leg, repeat steps 1, 2 & 3.

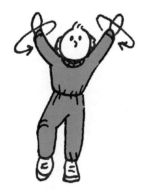

5.   Raise your right knee so your foot is just off the floor.
6.   Stretch your arms up in a "V" and trace small clockwise circles in the air.
7.   Lower your leg and arms and relax.
8.   Using your left leg, repeat steps 5, 6 & 7.

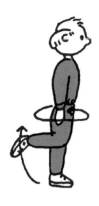

9. Bend your right leg at the knee so that your foot is behind you and just off the floor. Start with your arms hanging loosely at your sides. Then, gently trace small clockwise circles.

10. Lower leg and arms and relax.

11. Using your left leg, repeat steps 9 & 10.

REPETITIONS: 1 time, or as many as you enjoy!

A D V A N C E D   V E R S I O N

1. With arms in the various positions described previously (at shoulder level, in a "V," below shoulder level), try tracing circles in the air both clockwise and counterclockwise.

2. Once you've mastered the arms, try tracing simultaneous circles with your raised foot.

3. Now try tracing clockwise circles with your right hand while your left hand moves counter-clockwise. (It's like rubbing your tummy and patting your head at the same time.)

HOW TO PRACTICE FALLING
THE SAFE WAY

Have you ever practiced how to fall? Probably not. So when you do start to fall, you no doubt tense your body and become very rigid. (So does just about everybody, by the way!) That's why for just about everybody, the results of a fall can be very serious.

Now, no matter how careful you are, there will be times when an accidental fall may occur. So, be prepared for it! Prepared by training your body to remain loose and flexible--to be on **"automatic pilot,"** by having practiced maintaining and regaining your balance.

Your chair and your bed offer you very safe ways to practice falling down. Try it with **"Fall Out Shelter"** (both I & II), and you'll be better prepared to fall the safe way.

FALL OUT SHELTER
PART I – CHAIR

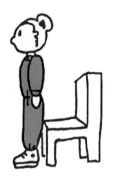

FOR STARTERS: Stand tall in front of your stationary chair, with the seat brushing the backs of your legs. Feet should be a comfortable distance apart and arms should be at your sides.

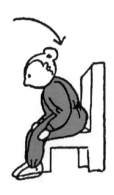

1. Totally relax your body and **s - l - o - w - l - y** let yourself **relax** and slump back into the chair.

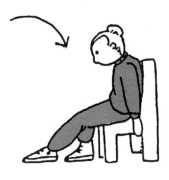

2. Slump your shoulders and do your best "rag doll" impression!

REPETITIONS: As often as possible. Have a contest with your friends. Who has the most relaxed "sit-down"?

FALL OUT SHELTER
PART II – BED

FOR STARTERS: Stand tall, feet comfortably apart with bed brushing the backs of your legs and arms hanging loosely at sides. You should be standing right in front of the **center** of your bed, with your back toward the bed.

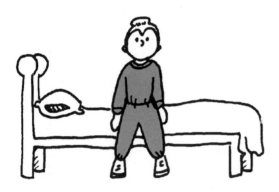

1. Bending at the knees, **s-l-o-w-l-y** and very loosely collapse into a sitting position on the bed. Slump your shoulders forward and relax your entire body during this simulated "fall."

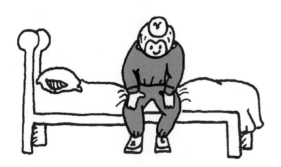

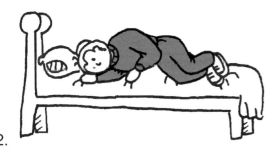

2.

2. Now, collapse on either your left shoulder and side or right shoulder and side (whichever is most comfortable for you), still staying as loose and limber as possible, bringing your knees up toward your chest in a semi-fetal position. (You will be lying down as shown in Figure 2.)

3. Return to starting position and repeat.

REPETITIONS: Every time you go to bed or lie down for a nap.

We will not have time to think "relax – let go." We must have trained our minds and bodies to fall loose. We must practice to be able to regain our balance if we start to "lose it" or to "fall like cooked spaghetti" if the need arises. We either practice and use our ability to maintain our balance or we lose it.

TAKE IT ALL IN STRIDE

We know that the risks of falling can be reduced by improving balance. We know that movement is the key to balance. And that muscle fitness contributes to movement. A good deal of movement relies on having strong, healthy feet and good leg muscles.

The more fit our feet and legs are, the more resistant we will be to falls. The muscles in our feet and legs provide the steady foundation on which our balancing activities are based.

One of the most efficient activities to promote the overall fitness of the body, and particularly the feet and toes, is walking. That's right, walking.

In my book, **The Fun of Fitness**, I have designed a number of walking activities which I think are important enough to include again here. Walking not only contributes to improvement in your cardiovascular system, it also acts as an overall toner and body strengthener. And, as if that weren't enough, 45 minutes of brisk walking can:

- work off about 300 calories (for a slimmer, trimmer you);
- improve your circulation and energy, endurance and elimination;
- improve your flexibility;
- reduce depression;
- counteract insomnia (a late afternoon or early evening walk is better than a sleeping pill);
- improve your social life (more about that later).

WORK ON WALKING

Here are a few tips on making the most out of walking. And, just like our formal activities section, they start with warming up!

Before you go for a walk or try any walking "variations," be sure to warm up your legs a little. You could start with either or both of these calf muscle stretcher/strengtheners.

JUST LEANING AROUND

1. With your back straight and your feet together, stand arm's length away from a wall.
2. Bend your elbows so your forearms "lean" against the wall (or, if you prefer, so that your bent elbows are out to the sides like "wings").
3. Hold the bent arm position for 5 to 10 seconds. (Remember to keep your heels flat on the floor!)
4. Relax and repeat as often as you feel necessary. (Some people find they like doing this exercise in the morning, again at noon and then just before going to bed at night.)

> Get off the bus early and walk!
> Walk to the store!
> Wear out the rugs right at home!
> Use the stairs!
> (Start with one flight then gradually climb more)
> Substitute a quick walk down the block for one of your favorite (too rich) desserts!

WARM UP FIRST!
You'll avoid shin splints and strained heel cords.

JAMB SESSION

This warm-up is an ideal way to alleviate leg cramping!

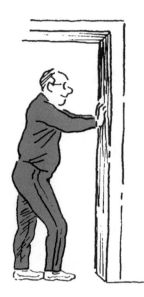

1. With your feet together, stand in front of a door jamb (arm's length away).
2. Holding onto the jamb, place your left foot directly behind your right (with toes of left foot touching heel of right foot and left heel flat on the floor).
3. Now, bend your right knee slightly and feel the stretch. Hold for a count of 1 – 2 – 3 – 4 – 5.
4. Straighten and return to starting position.
5. Relax, then repeat with other leg (2 times, total, with each leg).

No matter what your "stride" or walking pattern, there are just a couple more pointers (in addition to warming up) that can make walking work even better for you.

DRESS COMFORTABLY

- Especially if you're walking outdoors. You may want to dress in "layers," so that as you build up body heat you can take off a sweater or jacket, etc. along the way. On cold days, always wear a hat (to prevent too much loss of body heat).
- Wear comfortable, flat shoes. Sneakers or

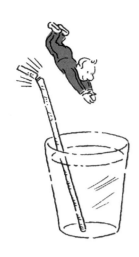

running shoes with a good arch support are your best bets. (Make sure they're not too tight, because your feet can swell a little as you walk.)

- Turn your socks inside out so the seams (if there are any) don't chafe and cause discomfort. (Remember to keep your toenails trimmed, too, as they can also be a "sore spot" for walkers!)

CHOOSE THE BEST TIME

In warm climates or seasons, walking (or any other outdoor exercising) should be done during the coolest parts of the day – early morning or after sunset.

On hot, humid days, be sure to increase your fluid intake.

STAND UP STRAIGHT

- Good posture is vital to a good walk. So, stand tall with your head and body erect.
- As you're walking, pay attention to keeping your chin up (with your neck as high as you can comfortably make it), chest up and shoulders back (with your hips "in line" under your shoulders).
- Your knees should be relaxed and your abdomen should be pulled in (toward an imaginary wall behind you).

READY, SET, WALK!

Walking is an activity that doesn't really have to be "learned." And our normal, everyday walking pattern is the perfect way to get started on the road to fitness and better balance. There are so many opportunities to "build the benefits" of walking, from gradually increasing the frequency to increasing the pace. Here's an exercise we can do by ourselves or with others, outdoors in perfect weather, or even inside, when the weather's not-so-perfect.

After you've started walking, try adding some fun (and flexibility for your legs, ankles, feet & toes) with a few of the walking variations my husband Mike and I are doing. (I'll admit, people sometimes wonder what we're up to, but I'll bet their balance and muscle tone don't hold a candle to ours!) Here's one occasion when sidestepping is a dandy way to get ahead. Just be careful how far you go.

VARIATION #1
SIDESTEP THE ISSUE!

- Next time you're out (or in!) walking, stop and then go to the right with a sideways step (or slide). Start with your right, then bring your left foot to meet (and touch) it.

- Step – close – step – close, until you've reached the curb or wall or any other "barrier."
- Now, sidestep to the left, back onto the "path" and continue your regular walk.

VARIATION # 2
ACTING UP

Play it cool – people will definitely wonder whether you're a clever pantomimist or just stuck on some bubblegum!

- Walk as though your feet were on slippery ice or marbles.
- Now, walk as though you were being blown by the wind, then swaying in a gentle breeze.
- Next, walk as though someone's tickling you.
- Finally, walk as though you were "ploughing" through rough ocean water or navigating a very crooked street.

(Use your imagination! Every time you walk, spend a few minutes pretending you're negotiating some difficult "terrain." You'll vary your pace and have a good laugh, too--probably at some spectators' expense!)

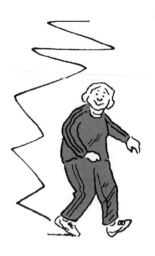

Walk in a zig-zag pattern…
Wiggle your body while you walk…
Walk like a robot…
Walk "heavy," then walk "light"…

VARIATION #3
TOE THE LINE

Here's another one where the forward progress isn't nearly as important as the strength you'll get in your calf muscles!

- Walk 8 steps forward on your "tiptoes," then 8 steps backward (still on your toes).
- Now, repeat these steps, but this time, lift your knees higher.
- "Toe the Line" as often as it feels good to you (or until someone complains that you're wearing out the rug)!

VARIATION # 4
GO TO THE HEAD OF THE CLASS!

An advanced variation for balance and overall leg strength and hip flexibility.

- On your tiptoes, swing right leg forward, then behind you once.
- Step onto right leg and swing left forward and behind.
- Repeat as often as is comfortable.

VARIATION # 5
SPRING FLING

I said "spring" because it rhymes! You can do this any season of the year.

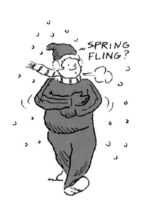

- As you walk, "fling" your arms across your chest, then out to the side in rhythmic repetitions.
- 8 flings (across and out) should do it every time you walk.

VARIATION # 6
SKATERS' WALTZ

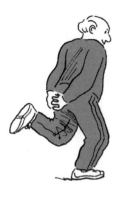

- Bring your arms comfortably behind your lower back, then clasp your hands together and stretch your arms as much as you can.
- Pull your arms down and back and walk in this position for 10 to 20 steps.
- Relax your arms – shake them loose, then repeat 2 or 3 times.

As soon as you try this you'll remember your smoothest glides across the ice.

GET IT TOGETHER!

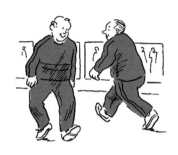

Walking is a great way to meet new people and enjoy the company of others who are as interested in fitness, better balance and fun as you are. One super place to find your contemporaries and have a regular, fun walk is in a shopping mall. (And for once you don't have to buy a thing!) In fact, lots of seniors now go to malls just to get in shape for walking.

What could be better, after all? Malls are climate-controlled, safe and spacious. (You can try all your variations there, too, and the worst you'll come up against is a wall!) Some malls open early for walkers. Others have clubs to bring walkers together.

However you plan your walk for health, don't waste another minute. Start now! Happy walking!

FITNOTE Stop by one of your own local malls and ask about their provisions for walking.

APPENDIX

Gain some control over your environment. Balance, movement and exercise help us to control some of the internal causes of falling, but we can all take the following simple steps to reduce the external risks of falling:

PROPER LIGHTING It is **very** important to have good lighting around your home.

1.   Always turn on lights before going into a room, even if you are only going in for a moment.
2.   Move slowly when lighting is dim. Give your eyes time to adjust before proceeding between well-lighted and dark areas.
3.   Replace any burned-out bulbs immediately; repair cords and fixtures.
4.   Night-lights are inexpensive and invaluable in contributing to visibility at night, particularly in stairwells, hallways, bathrooms and bedrooms. Night-lights or remote-control switches by the bedside are a good precaution. Keep a flashlight next to your bed in case of a power failure.
5.   Make sure indoor and outdoor walkways are properly illuminated, especially at night. Don't

overlook stairways, cellar areas, garages, storage rooms, or outdoor sheds. Have switches installed at both **top** and **bottom** of stairways.

6. On a bright day, or around ice or snow, wear sunglasses to reduce blinding glare.

7. A pull chain on a light is much easier to operate than other types of turn or push light switches.

SECURE WALKWAYS

1. Carpeting, particularly on stairs, provides additional cushioning to reduce the risk of injury if you should fall. In doorways, raised thresholds should be eliminated or covered with carpeting.

2. Carpeting should be securely fastened down with double-sided tape or carpet tacks. Repair holes in carpeting; get rid of frayed rugs; avoid throw rugs, as they can bunch up or slide. Skid-resistant rugs are available. If your rug has a non-skid backing, vacuum the backing often, because dirt keeps the non-skid finish from gripping the floor. (You can also tape rubber jar rings to the back of rugs to prevent them from sliding.)

3. Place bright, contrasting colored tape on the top and bottom steps of stairways. This serves as a constant reminder to BE CAREFUL. Change the colors periodically so

you won't become oblivious to the tape.

4. Keep walkways clear of miscellaneous or misplaced objects, especially electrical and telephone cords. Tape cords to the floor or wall; tie up extra cord with a rubber band, or coil it up inside an empty toilet paper tube. Place furniture over the edges of rugs to help hold them in place.

5. Replace small breaks in linoleum, broken floorboards or flooring that is buckling or warping so no one will trip over loose edges. Repair any furniture that is unsteady.

6. Don't take shortcuts off established walkways; they can be dangerous. Take the pathway provided and make sure you can see where you are going.

7. Be alert to pets and children who can pop up in front of or behind you.

8. Clean up all spills immediately, because a foot can slip easily on even a little spill, a little food on the floor or a grease spot.

9. To make walking safer in darkness, arrange your furniture in each room so that a lane is kept open.

BATHE SAFELY

1. Install and use tightly fastened grab bars in the bath tub, and on the wall next to the tub or shower, when possible. Enter and exit a shower or tub slowly and carefully. Securely

carpet all surfaces that might get wet or slippery.

2. Install non-slip strips or non-skid mats in bath tub or shower. (Now there are non-slip treatments available for bath tubs and floors.)

3. Grab bars or handrails can be installed by the toilet, and a higher-than-normal toilet seat is helpful. There are also handrail units that fit over the toilet and provide support, but do not have to be secured to the wall.)

4. Always test the tub or shower water to make sure it is not too hot, so that you do not make a quick reactive movement and lose your balance.

5. Sit on the side of the tub while lifting legs into the tub. When leaving the tub, make sure one foot is firmly on the floor and you feel in balance before lifting the other foot out.

6. Use a flexible shower hose. A hand-held shower can make bathing easier.

7. If you splash soap suds or drop a bar of soap, wipe up the floor right away.

8. As an extra precaution, you can dry yourself off before getting out of the tub.

SECURE HANDGRIPS

1. Install and use secure handrails on **both** sides of the stairways, running their full length. If you should start to fall, do not let go of the railing: **hang on**.

FOOTWEAR

1. Wear footwear with soles and heels that provide good support and traction between your feet and the surface you walk on, especially when you venture on to snow or ice. **Friction helps prevent falls.**

2. Keep the soles of your shoes clean and free of any oil or mud that might accumulate on them.

3. Avoid wearing only socks or smooth-soled shoes or slippers on stairs, wood or waxed floors. They make it easy to slip.

WET, SLIPPERY OR UNFAMILIAR, UNEVEN SURFACES

1. Choose shoes and overshoes that have slip-resistant soles.

2. Point your feet outward slightly, and maintain a steady pace.

3. Make wide turns when you are going around corners.

4. Pay attention to the surface you are walking on: be alert for ice, snow, wet or dry leaves, moss-covered stone paths or steps.

5. Keep your hands out of your pockets, and free to help you with better balance. If you have to carry a bag of groceries, make sure your other hand is free.

6. Remember to salt icy sidewalks and pathways.

7. When you get out of a car, test the condition of the ground for wetness or iciness before standing up and walking. Don't hurry--be wary!

8. When walking on slippery or uneven surfaces, lean forward slightly, relax your knees, and take shorter steps to keep your center of balance under you. You may prefer to "shuffle" your steps, keeping each foot flat on the ground. Falls occur whenever you move too far off your center of balance. Tripping, for example, can push you off your center of balance far enough to cause a fall.

GENERAL SAFETY

1. When coming down steps, **feel** the back of your leg against the step so you won't slip off. Put your whole foot down and **concentrate** on each movement as you descend the stairs.

2. When you visit friends, be alert to possible hazards, as you are in an unfamiliar environment; you may even be able to alert friends to any problems that they are unaware of in their homes. Be especially careful of stepped entrances and elevations in split-level homes.

3. Curbs can be dangerous. Some are poorly identified, broken, very high, and sometimes badly illuminated. Be alert as you enter and exit any areas that have curbs. It is so easy to be talking to a friend, and not be alert to danger.

4. Carts in a supermarket can also be a problem. Do not walk backwards even 1, 2, or

3 feet to reach for that can of tuna fish you forgot as it is too easy to lose your balance and fall backward. Take the extra few minutes to go around the aisle.

5. Let the phone ring--don't run to answer it. Your friends will call again. And make sure the phone is convenient to the bed, easily reached.

6. Never, never climb on a chair to change a light bulb or to reach a high shelf or cabinet. If you must reach a high shelf, use a sturdy stepladder.

PERSONAL ETCs.

1. Have your vision and hearing tested regularly and properly corrected. Even the simple task of removing ear wax can improve your balance.

2. Use caution in getting up too quickly after eating, lying down or resting. Low blood pressure may cause dizziness at these times.

3. Talk to your doctor or pharmacist about the side effects of the drugs you are taking and how they may affect your coordination or balance.

4. Limit your intake of alcohol. Even a little alcohol can further disturb already impaired balance and reflexes.

5. Make sure that the nighttime temperature in your home is not lower than 65°F. Prolonged

exposure to cold temperatures may cause body temperatures to drop, leading to dizziness and falling. Many older persons cannot tolerate cold as well as younger people can.

6. Use a cane, walking stick, or walker to help maintain balance on uneven or unfamiliar ground or if you sometimes feel dizzy. Use special caution in walking outdoors on wet and icy pavement.

7. Maintain a regular program of activity. Many people enjoy walking, swimming and exercise. Mild weight-bearing activities may reduce the loss of bone from osteoporosis. It is important, however, to check with your doctor or physical therapist to plan a suitable exercise program.

AFTERWORD

I think we've covered a number of important issues in this booklet. We have known for some time that the fear and real dangers of falling have been leading causes of forced inactivity among our ever-growing senior population, **but** we are just discovering that that no longer needs to be true. We **can** take charge of our own lives. By conquering our fear and by practicing The Balance System activities, we can actually minimize the risks involved in falling.

As I described earlier, I've seen remarkable changes in every one of my senior students. And what has been true for them can be true for you! All it takes is your determination and your commitment to setting and achieving your goals.

Remember, the benefits to be gained from making The Balance System part of your daily routine go far beyond preventing many falls. Movement and exercise decrease the problems associated with such physical disorders as arthritis, osteoporosis, high blood pressure and heart disease, among others. In addition, they also enhance your mental, emotional and social well-being. How can you go wrong?

Age is not a factor. You **can** exercise some control over the quality of your life. So, start today!

ORDER FORM

☎ **Telephone orders:** Call Toll Free **1-800-525-3707.** (9-5 M-F Eastern Time for MasterCard and Visa.)

How To Prevent Falls – $9.95 plus $2.00 postage and handling per book
The Fun of Fitness – $16.95 plus $3.00 postage and handling per book
(both books – $22.95 plus $5.00 postage and handling)

Please send _____ **copies of** *How To Prevent Falls*
Please send _____ **copies of** *The Fun of Fitness*

Fill out other side and send with check or money order to:
Senior Fitness Productions, Inc., Betty Perkins-Carpenter
P.O. Box 25413
Rochester, New York 14625-2394 USA   *(over)*

ORDER FORM

☎ **Telephone orders:** Call Toll Free **1-800-525-3707.** (9-5 M-F Eastern Time for MasterCard and Visa.)

How To Prevent Falls – $9.95 plus $2.00 postage and handling per book
The Fun of Fitness – $16.95 plus $3.00 postage and handling per book
(both books – $22.95 plus $5.00 postage and handling)

Please send _____ **copies of** *How To Prevent Falls*
Please send _____ **copies of** *The Fun of Fitness*

Fill out other side and send with check or money order to:
Senior Fitness Productions, Inc., Betty Perkins-Carpenter
P.O. Box 25413
Rochester, New York 14625-2394   *(over)*

ORDER FORM

☎ **Telephone orders:** Call Toll Free **1-800-525-3707.** (9-5 M-F Eastern Time for MasterCard and Visa.)

How To Prevent Falls – $9.95 plus $2.00 postage and handling per book
The Fun of Fitness – $16.95 plus $3.00 postage and handling per book
(both books – $22.95 plus $5.00 postage and handling)

Please send _____ **copies of** *How To Prevent Falls*
Please send _____ **copies of** *The Fun of Fitness*

Fill out other side and send with check or money order to:
Senior Fitness Productions, Inc., Betty Perkins-Carpenter
P.O. Box 25413
Rochester, New York 14625-2394 USA   *(over)*

☐ Please add my name to your mailing list so that I may receive more information on balance activities.

Name _____

Address _____

City _____ State _____ Zip _____

Payment: ☐ Check   ☐ Money order   Amount enclosed _____

New York residents only – add 7% sales tax.

Call toll free and order now! 1-800-525-3707
(9-5 M-F Eastern Time for MasterCard and Visa.)

☐ Please add my name to your mailing list so that I may receive more information on balance activities.

Name _____

Address _____

City _____ State _____ Zip _____

Payment: ☐ Check   ☐ Money order   Amount enclosed _____

New York residents only – add 7% sales tax.

Call toll free and order now! 1-800-525-3707
(9-5 M-F Eastern Time for MasterCard and Visa.)

☐ Please add my name to your mailing list so that I may receive more information on balance activities.

Name _____

Address _____

City _____ State _____ Zip _____

Payment: ☐ Check   ☐ Money order   Amount enclosed _____

New York residents only – add 7% sales tax.

Call toll free and order now! 1-800-525-3707
(9-5 M-F Eastern Time for MasterCard and Visa.)